Body Butter Essentials

A Guide For Making Your Own Luxurious Body Butter

Disclaimer and Terms of Use:

Effort has been made to ensure that the information in this book is accurate and complete, however, the author and the publisher do not warrant the accuracy of the information, text and graphics contained within the book due to the rapidly changing nature of science, research, known and unknown facts and internet. The Author and the publisher do not hold any responsibility for errors, omissions or contrary interpretation of the subject matter herein. This book is presented solely for motivational and informational purposes only.

Table of Contents

Introduction

Body butter is a moisturizer that softens, hydrates and rejuvenates skin. It is somewhat similar to lotion, but is thicker, with yogurt-like texture. Body butters usually uses Cocoa butter, Shea butter, Coconut Oil or other vegetable-based oils as a base.

It is best used for the body to hydrate and protect the skin. Body butter is especially effective for softening and rejuvenating problem areas such as the elbows, knees and feet. After shaving your legs and underarms, apply body butter to prevent drying and to keep them moisturized.

Body butter is a staple beauty product for both men and women. With just a small amount, you will get a rich and creamy lather with body butter. It is much more effective in keeping the skin hydrated all day. Furthermore, body butters contain ingredients that are very nourishing to the skin such cocoa beans, Shea nuts, Kukui nut and mango seeds. These ingredients are full of nutrients that effectively nourish the skin.

Aside from keeping your skin moisturized, body butters also protect your skin by forming a protective barrier which holds in moisture. Therefore, your skin stays hydrated even under the sun or during cold winter. In addition, body butters are very affordable.

Keep on reading to learn more about how to make your own body butter that suits your skin well.

Chapter 1   Tools And Ingredients For Making Body Butter

The tools needed for making body butter is pretty basic. You can find most of them in your kitchen.

You will need the following tools:

a) Mixing bowl

b) Electric beater or whisker

c) Measuring cups

d) Measuring spoons

e) Sterile container

The basic ingredients for body butter are:

a) Plant butter – Shea butter, Cocoa butter, Mango butter,   etc.

b) Oils – Jojoba oil, Coconut oil, Almond Oil, Grapeseed Oil, Soy Oil, Avocado Oil and others

c) Essential Oil – any fragrance to your liking

But, before you start, remember these safety tips:

1. Wear kitchen apron to keep your clothes from getting stained and burned while working.

2. Kitchen gloves are a must to prevent your hands and skin from too much heat and burning.

3. Your working area should have a flat surface to prevent spilling while mixing your materials.

Making your own body butter is very easy, but you need to keep those tips in mind to keep safe.

Chapter 2   25 Body Butter Recipes You Can Do At Home

1. Basic Shea Body Butter Recipe

Ingredients:

1 1/3 cups ultra-refined Shea Butter

½ cup Olive Oil

1 teaspoon Vitamin E Oil

½ oz. pure Lavender Essential Oil

Directions:

1. Slowly melt the Shea butter in a double broiler. You can do this in a stove top but make sure the heat is on low.

2. Add olive oil when Shea butter is completely melted. Mix thoroughly.

3. Set aside for 30 minutes to cool. Add Vitamin E oil and Lavender essential oil. Whip with a hand mixer until it becomes like whipped cream. If consistency is not setting up, place in the refrigerator for 10 minutes before whipping again.

4. Store in a clean, wide-mouth container with lid.

2. Jojoba Oil Body Butter

Ingredients:

10 oz ultra-refined Shea Butter

¾ cup Jojoba Oil

2 teaspoons Cornstarch

10 drops Orange Essential Oil

5 drops Mandarin Essential Oil

5 drops Vanilla Essential Oil

Directions:

1. Melt Shea butter until it turns into liquid.

2. Remove from heat. Add Jojoba oil, essential oils and cornstarch. Mix until well blended.

3. Chill the pan in a bowl full of ice. Watch out for the water on the sides as they may go over the pan and ruin your body butter.

4. With an electric hand mixer, beat until soft peaks form.

5. Store in a clean wide-mouth container with lid.

3. Chamomile Lavender Body Butter

Ingredients:

10 oz Shea Butter

6 oz Jojoba Oil

10 drops Chamomile Essential Oil

10 drops Lavender Essential Oil

2 tablespoons Cornstarch

Directions:

1. Melt the Shea butter in a double broiler. You may also use a heatproof bowl and place it in a pan of boiling water. When Shea butter is already soft and can be mixed easily with a spoon, remove from heat and add Jojoba oil. Mix well.

2. Stir in essential oils and cornstarch. Transfer to a mixing bowl and beat with and electric hand mixer or process in a blender.

3. Mix until consistency is like whipped cream and peaks form. That's about 10 minutes. Mix for another 10 minutes if consistency is not yet achieved.

4. Transfer the body butter into clean decorative glasses with tight-fitting lids.

4. Aloe Vera Body Butter

Ingredients:

½ cup Cocoa Butter

½ cup Shea Butter

¼ cup Aloe Vera gel

3 tablespoon grated Beeswax

1 teaspoon Vanilla Extract

Directions:

1. Melt beeswax with ¼ cup water in a double broiler. Mix vigorously until it melts. Keep warm.

2. Melt Cocoa butter and Shea butter together in the double broiler. Remove from heat as soon as the butters are soft and can be easily mixed. Avoid cooking the butters.

3. Combine melted beeswax, vanilla extract and Aloe Vera gel in the melted butters. Mix the ingredients using a hand-held blender until you get a thick and creamy consistency.

4. Store in dry, clean containers with wide mouth and tight lid. Refrigerate when not in use to prolong shelf life up to three months.

5. Mango Cocoa Body Butter

Ingredients:

½ cup Shea butter

½ cup Cocoa butter

½ cup Mango butter

¾ cup Apricot Kernel oil

¾ cup Wheat Germ oil

3 tablespoons Beeswax pearls

20 drops Mango essential oil

2 teaspoons Vitamin E oil

Directions:

1. Place the Shea butter, Cocoa butter, Mango butter, Apricot Kernel oil, Wheat Germ oil and beeswax in a microwave safe bowl.

2. Melt the mixture one batch at a time until all ingredients have completely melted. Set the microwave on low and heat it for 2 to 3 minutes. Do not boil.

3. Once melted, stir until all ingredients are well combined.

4. Let it cool for a few hours and stir again.

5. Make sure to stir in the Mango essential oil before the mixture sets.

6. Store Mango body butter in a jar or tin and keep in a cool, dark place. You may also refrigerate to prolong shelf life.

6. Creamy Mocha Body Butter

Ingredients:

2 oz. Cocoa butter

2 oz. Shea butter

1 teaspoon Aloe Vera gel

3 teaspoons Apricot Kernel oil

¼ teaspoon French Vanilla fragrance oil

¼ teaspoon Coffee fragrance oil

¼ teaspoon Chocolate fragrance oil

Directions:

1. In a double boiler, liquefy Cocoa butter and Shea butter on low heat. Keep mixing until the butters are completely melted. Simmer for 20 minutes but do not allow boiling.

2. Pour in a bowl and mix with an electric hand mixer or mix in a blender. Add Apricot Kernel oil while mixture is still warm. Mix until well blended and allow cooling for about 10 minutes or less.

3. Add Aloe Vera gel and Vitamin E. Beat with electric mixer until well blended.

4. Mix all the fragrance oils in a bowl and add it into the butter mixture. Blend until you reach a mousse-like consistency.

5. Store in a clean, dry container with air-tight lid.

7. Vanilla Bean Body Butter Cream

Ingredients:

1 cup Cocoa Butter

½ cup Coconut oil

½ cup Sweet Almond oil

1 Vanilla bean

Directions:

1. Melt coconut oil and cocoa butter. Stir and let cool for about 30 minutes.

2. Using a coffee grinder or food processor, grind the vanilla bean and mix it in the coconut oil and cocoa butter mixture. Add sweet almond oil and mix thoroughly.

3. Chill in the freezer for 20 minutes or until oil starts to solidify.

4. Blend in a food processor or whip using an electric mixer until the consistency is that of butter.

5. Transfer in a glass jar using a spoon. Glass container is advisable due to the essential oils which can absorb toxins from plastic containers.

8. Easy Coconut Oil Body Butter

Ingredients:

1 cup Coconut oil

1 teaspoon Vitamin E oil

10 drops Rose essential oil

10 drops Vanilla essential oil

Directions:

1. Combine all ingredients in a mixing bowl. Do not melt the coconut oil as it won't whip when it is liquefied.

2. Whisk with an electric mixer until you get an airy, light consistency.

3. Transfer coconut oil body butter in a clean container with a tight lid and store in room temperature. To prevent the oil from melting, store in refrigerator.

9. Avocado Body Butter

Ingredients:

9 oz. Cocoa butter

9 oz. Avocado oil

20 drops Lavender essential oil

15 drops Chamomile essential oil

15 drops Geranium essential oil

3 teaspoons Cornstarch

Directions:

1. Melt the Cocoa butter in a double broiler in medium heat until soft enough to be stirred easily. Be careful not to overheat.

2. Stir in Avocado oil, essential oils and cornstarch. Ingredients must be thoroughly blended.

3. Cool the mixture in a bowl of ice water.

4. Whip with an electric mixer until it has the consistency of a whipped cream and stiff peaks form.

5. Spoon avocado body butter into clean jars. You may refrigerate for longer shelf life but it will have a firmer consistency.

10. Whipped Body Butter Cream

Ingredients:

½ cup Shea butter

¼ cup Jojoba oil

¼ cup Coconut oil

5 drops Peppermint essential oil

5 drops Eucalyptus essential oil

Directions:

1. In a glass bowl or measuring cup placed inside a saucepan with water, place the Coconut oil, Jojoba oil and Shea butter to melt. Make sure the saucepan has enough water in it but should not spill out. Heat over medium temperature.

2. Mix the oils until they are melted and well-combined. When mixture becomes white or semi-clear, it is ready.

3. Refrigerate the mixture until solid and white.

4. With a hand mixer or stand mixer, whisk the oil mixture until it reaches the consistency of a whipped cream. Add essential oils and whisk with mixer to incorporate.

5. Transfer into clean, dry glass jars and refrigerate for 1 hour. This body butter may soften during hot weather. If so, store in refrigerator.

11. Peppermint Tallow Body Butter

Ingredients:

½ cup Tallow

½ cup Jojoba oil

1 cup Shea butter

1 teaspoon Peppermint essential oil

2 teaspoons Vitamin E oil

Directions:

1. Heat Tallow and Shea butter until melted. You can use a double broiler or a glass bowl placed on top of a pot with simmering water.

2. Once melted, remove from heat and stir in Jojoba oil. Chill in an ice bath or a bowl full of ice water for 5 minutes. Mix in the Peppermint essential oil and Vitamin E oil. Continue to chill in the ice bath until completely cool.

3. Using an electric mixer (hand or stand mixer), whip the mixture until soft peaks form or until it reaches the consistency of a whipped cream.

4. Spoon into airtight container and keep away from sunlight. Store in dark, dry area. This body butter can last up to a year if stored properly.

12. Tea Tree Body Butter

Ingredients:

6 tablespoons Cocoa butter

2 tablespoons Jojoba oil

½ cup Coconut oil

2 tablespoons Vitamin E oil

20 drops Tea Tree oil

15 drops Lavender oil

Directions:

1. Melt the cocoa butter at low temperature and remove from heat as soon as it's melted.

2. Stir in coconut oil and Jojoba oil until the coconut oil is fully melted.

3. Wait for the mixture to solidify. You can wait 24 hours at room temperature or place in the refrigerator.

4. Whip solidified mixture using a stand or hand mixer on high.

5. Stir in tea tree oil and mix until double in volume.

6. Scoop into glass jars with airtight lids.

13. Luxurious Peppermint Body Butter

Ingredients:

½ cup Cocoa butter

½ cup Shea butter

½ cup Coconut oil

½ cup Sweet Almond oil

1 teaspoon Vitamin E oil

4 drops Peppermint essential oils

Directions:

1. In a medium pot, combine Coconut oil, Cocoa butter and Shea butter over low heat. Mix until oils are completely melted and remove from heat.

2. Stir in Sweet Almond oil, Vitamin E oil and essential oil. Mix thoroughly.

3. Place in the refrigerator for one to two hours or until mixture is firm but not very hard.

4. Once the mixture is chilled, mix using a hand or stand mixer until you reach a whipped cream consistency. Scoop into a container and store in dark, dry area. This body butter cream can last up to 12 months at room temperature. If it melts, just re-chill and whip it again.

14. Citrus Mango Body Butter

Ingredients:

½ cup Mango butter

½ cup Shea butter

½ cup Coconut oil

½ cup Almond oil or Jojoba oil

10 drops Mandarin essential oil

10 drops Orange essential oil

10 drops Lemon essential oil

Directions:

1. Combine all ingredients in a double broiler or a glass bowl in simmering water. Melt the ingredients while constantly mixing. Remove from heat when completely melted.

2. Let cool for a few minutes and chill in the refrigerator for 1 hour or until the mixture is set but not too hard.

3. Whip using a hand or stand mixer until you get a fluffy consistency.

4. Put the body butter back in the refrigerator to set for about 10 to 15 minutes.

5. Store in a glass container. Keep in the fridge if temperature in your house gets warm to keep it whipped.

15. Relaxing Magnesium Body Butter

Ingredients:

½ cup Magnesium flakes

3 tablespoons boiling Water

¼ cup unrefined Coconut oil

2 tablespoons Beeswax Pastilles

3 tablespoons Shea butter

Directions:

1. In a small bowl, mix together 3 tablespoons of boiling water and magnesium flakes. Mix until completely dissolved and liquid becomes thick. Set aside.

2. In a glass bowl placed in a pan with water, combine Shea butter, Coconut oil and Beeswax Pastilles. Melt over medium heat.

3. Remove from heat and let it cool at room temperature. When mixture is already cool or slightly opaque, transfer in a bowl and mix with hand-held blender. You can also use a blender or stand mixer.

4. Add the dissolve magnesium into the oil mixture one drop at a time while blending. Continue to blend until all the magnesium is added and thoroughly mixed.

5. Chill in the fridge for 15 minutes. Blend one more time to get a whipped cream consistency. Store in the fridge when not in use for best consistency.

16. Anti-Cellulite Body Butter Cream

Ingredients:

50 grams Shea butter

50 grams Cocoa butter

100 grams Coconut oil

30 drops Cinnamon essential oil

A few Cinnamon sticks

Directions:

1. Warm Cocoa butter and Shea butter in a pan in low heat until it turns liquid.

2. Stir in the Coconut oil and turn off heat. Cool for 10 to 20 minutes in room temperature. Do not refrigerate to allow gentle setting.

3. Add the Cinnamon oil as soon as the mixture cools. Whip it until consistency becomes fluffy and light.

4. Break the Cinnamon sticks into pieces and add to the mixture. Mix one more time to blend cinnamon sticks thoroughly into the mixture.

5. Store in air-tight container.

17. Easy Coco Honey Body Butter

Ingredients:

1 ½ cups solid Coconut oil

3 tablespoons Honey

2 tablespoons zest of Grapefruit, Lemon or Orange

Directions:

1. Combine all ingredients in a bowl and whisk with an electric mixer until smooth and fluffy.

2. Store in a tightly closed container and keep in the refrigerator when not in use.

3. This body butter cream can only last for a week or two and is best used as shaving cream for the legs and moisturizer in problem areas.

18. Citrus Honey Body Butter

Ingredients:

2 tablespoons Beeswax

½ cup Grapeseed oil

1 capsule Vitamin E oil

3 tablespoons Distilled Water

10 drops Lemon essential oil

Directions:

1. Combine the Beeswax, Grapeseed oil and Vitamin E oil. Heat until the beeswax is just about melted.

2. Beat the warm oils using a hand mixer and add the distilled water little by little while mixing. Mix until mixture becomes milky.

3. Add the lemon essential oil and mix until it becomes smooth and fluffy.

4. Allow to sit for 15 to 20 minutes to set before scooping into an air-tight container. This body butter can last up to two months in room temperature. It can last longer if kept in the refrigerator.

19. Body Butter Cream For Sensitive Skin

Ingredients:

90 grams Shea butter

45 grams Cocoa butter

45 grams Kukui Nut oil

20 drops Spearmint essential oil

10 drops Rosemary essential oil

Directions:

1. In a glass or metal bowl, combine the Cocoa butter, Shea butter and Kukui oil.

2. Place in a pan of simmering water and melt butters over medium-low heat.

3. Allow to cool in room temperature and chill in the fridge for 20 minutes.

4. Blend with a hand mixer until mixture becomes white and creamy.

5. Return in the fridge until cold. Keep whisking until fluffy. Add essential oils and blend again until you reach the consistency of a whipped cream. This body butter cream lasts up to 30 days but longer if kept in the fridge.

20. Skin Conditioning Body Butter Cream

Ingredients:

4 tablespoons Coconut oil

3 tablespoons Aloe Vera gel

2 tablespoons Beeswax

1.5 tablespoons Olive oil

2 teaspoons Lanolin

1 teaspoon Honey

1 capsule Vitamin E

10 drops Lavender essential oil

Directions:

1. Heat Coconut oil, Olive oil and Beeswax over medium heat in a double broiler or pot with simmering water.

2. In a separate bowl, melt Aloe gel and mix into the oil mixture.

3. Stir in Lanolin until melted. Remove from heat. Mix Vitamin E and Lavender essential oil.

4. Whip with electric mixer until smooth and creamy.

5. Transfer into glass jars and cool in the fridge for 10 minutes before covering for best consistency.

21. Coco-Vanilla Body Butter Cream

Ingredients:

½ cup Shea butter

¼ cup Coconut oil

1 tablespoon Vitamin E oil

½ teaspoon Vanilla oil

Directions:

1. Place a heat-resistant bowl on top of a pot with boiling water.

2. Put the Shea butter in the bowl. While it's melting, add the coconut oil. Stir until completely melted.

3. Stir in Vanilla oil and Vitamin E oil. Transfer in a container with cover and chill in the freezer for 10 minutes.

4. Whip with a hand mixer until creamy and color is somewhat white. It should be smooth and creamy.

5. Spoon into clean and dry container with air-tight lid. This body butter cream is great as a moisturizer for underarms and legs after shaving.

22. Sensual Chocolate Body Butter

Ingredients:

¾ cup Coconut oil

1/3 cup Agave nectar

½ tablespoon Vanilla powder

¼ cup Cacao powder

2 drops Rose essential oil

½ teaspoon powdered Lavender flowers

Directions:

1. Melt Coconut oil and add Cacao powder, Vanilla powder and Agave nectar. Mix well with a hand mixer until thick and creamy.

2. Add Rose essential oil and powdered Lavender flowers. Mix until smooth and all ingredients are well incorporated.

3. Pour into clean, dry containers and chill in the fridge to set. Store in a cool, dry place.

23. Scentfully Luxurious Black Raspberry Body Butter

Ingredients:

156 grams Cocoa butter

155 grams Shea butter

65 grams Apricot Kernel oil

24 grams Grapeseed oil

10 grams Black Raspberry Vanilla fragrance oil

4 grams Vitamin E oil

Directions:

1. Using the double boiler method, melt the butters and add Grapeseed oil and Apricot Kernel oil. Stir until completely melted but be careful not to overheat.

2. Remove from heat and add fragrance oil. Mix until well combined.

3. Let cool in room temperature and chill in the fridge to set. Once cool, mix with an electric mixer until thick. Put mixture back into the fridge and allow cooling again. Whip until it looks like whipped butter. Repeat the process until the mixture is solid enough and no longer runny.

4. Place in clean, dry jars with air-tight cover. You can store it in the fridge when not in use to keep consistency and prolong shelf life.

24. Rose Coconut Body Butter Cream

Ingredients:

1 cup Coconut oil

½ cup Shea butter

1 tablespoon Vitamin E oil

10 drops Rose essential oil

Directions:

1. Melt the Shea butter using the double boiler method. While it's melting, stir in the Coconut oil.

2. When completely melted, remove from heat and transfer to a clean container. Allow to cool in room temperature then put in the freezer for 10 minutes.

3. Mix with hand mixer until white and creamy. Add Vitamin E oil and essential oil. Mix until it reaches the consistency of a whipped cream.

4. Transfer in containers with tight lids. Store in the fridge when not in use for better consistency and prolonged shelf life.

25. Almond Coconut Shea Body Butter

Ingredients:

¼ cup Almond oil

¼ cup Coconut oil

½ cup Shea butter

10 drops Lavender essential oil

5 drops Rose essential oil

Directions:

1. Mix all ingredients and heat them using the double boiler method. Stir until all ingredients are melted.

2. Transfer in a container and cool in room temperature for an hour. You can also place it in the fridge if you want it to set faster.

3. As soon as the oils are solid on the edges, whip with an electric mixer until soft peaks start to form and the mixture looks like whipped cream.

4. Place in a clean, dry container with a tight lid and store in a dark, cool place.

Chapter 3   Benefits Of Body Butter Creams

Body butter creams offer a lot of benefits to the skin. The ingredients used in making body butter creams contain healing qualities, anti-inflammatory properties and antioxidant content that helps nourish and protect skin from damage.

Shea butter contains fatty acids that helps heal the skin. It also helps heal swelling tissues and contains Vitamin A and E as well as antioxidants that prevent the skin from damage due to UV radiation.

Cocoa butter contains high fatty acids and effectively hydrates skin. It also contains antioxidants that fights off free radicals that causes stress and aging.

Coconut oil improves lipid content and moisture in the skin. It also blocks about 20% of UV rays from the sun, making it an effective natural sunscreen. Plus, coconut oil contains a combination of fatty acids that has very powerful medicinal properties.

Jojoba oil is rich in Vitamin E that helps reduce scars, stretch marks and scabs. It also helps boost the healing process of wounds. Jojoba oil also reduces skin dryness and irritation.

Essentials oils, on the other hand, are known for their therapeutic effects. Essential oils are commonly used for relaxation and as a mood enhancer. There are various essential oils that you can choose from, depending on your needs.

In other words, body butter creams are good food for the skin. They keep your skin moisturized, smooth, soft and hydrated for a long time. Body butter creams are great especially for the elbows, knees, bikini line and feet. Body butter creams that contain Jojoba oil and Coconut oil are also used by some for a softer, more manageable hair.

Conclusion

Making your own body butter cream is not at all that hard. The tools you need are already in your kitchen and the ingredients are easy to find in the market.

Furthermore, you can control what goes into your body butter cream and choose the ingredients that work best for your skin. You can make your own body butter cream and share it with your friends.

It is also very practical and economical to make your own body butter cream. Commercial body butter creams costs around $20 to $30 dollars per bottle or container. But, if you make your own body butter cream, you can already make 3 to 4 jars with the price of one commercial body butter cream.

It is also important to note that homemade body butter creams are preservative-free, so there is lesser chance of toxins getting in your body. For healthier living, going natural is the way to go.

Mix and match the ingredients until you come up with one that suits your body well. You can substitute the oils used in the recipes to conform to your needs.

Next thing you know, you are already distributing body butter creams to your friends, family and neighbors.

Enjoy this book?

Please leave a review below and let us know what you liked about this book.